The PCOS Diet Cookbook

The PCOS Diet Cookbook

Take Control of Your PCOS with Easy Meal Prep & Over 75 Recipes for Women Managing Polycystic Ovarian Syndrome on the Insulin Resistance Diet

Lila Thompson

The PCOS Foodie

Hopliv Publisher

CONTENTS

Introduction

Overview of PCOS and Insulin Resistance

Polycystic Ovarian Syndrome (PCOS) is a condition that affects millions of women worldwide. It's not just about irregular periods or fertility issues—PCOS can influence many aspects of a woman's health, from her weight to her skin, and even her mood. The culprit? Often, it's insulin resistance.

Insulin resistance is when your body doesn't respond well to insulin, a hormone that helps control blood sugar levels. When your cells resist insulin, your body produces more of it, which can lead to a variety of health issues, including PCOS. This is why managing insulin resistance through diet is crucial for women with PCOS.

Purpose of the Cookbook

This cookbook is designed to help you manage your PCOS symptoms through delicious, easy-to-make meals that support insulin sensitivity. We know how overwhelming it can be to balance life with the demands of a special diet, so we've focused on recipes that are not only healthy but also simple and enjoyable to prepare.

Personal Anecdote

My journey with PCOS began in my early twenties. I remember the confusion and frustration, the countless doctor visits, and the never-ending search for answers. One day, a friend introduced me to the concept of managing PCOS through diet. At first, it seemed impossible —another thing to add to my already overflowing plate. But then, I started seeing changes: my energy levels improved, my mood stabilized, and for the first time in years, I felt in control.

This cookbook is my way of sharing that discovery with you. I want to make it easier for you to find joy in cooking, even when dealing with PCOS. So, let's get started—one delicious meal at a time.

Understanding PCOS and Insulin Resistance

What is PCOS?

PCOS, or Polycystic Ovarian Syndrome, is a hormonal disorder common among women of reproductive age. It can cause prolonged or infrequent menstrual periods, excess androgen levels, and polycystic ovaries. The name itself can be misleading; not all women with PCOS have cysts on their ovaries, but the syndrome can still wreak havoc on their bodies.

Symptoms and Diagnosis

- **Symptoms:** Irregular periods, excessive hair growth, acne, obesity, and infertility.
- **Diagnosis:** Often diagnosed through a combination of medical history, physical exams, blood tests to measure hormone levels, and ultrasound to check for ovarian cysts.

Common Misconceptions

- **Myth:** PCOS only affects overweight women. **Fact:** Women of all sizes can have PCOS.

- **Myth:** You can't get pregnant if you have PCOS. **Fact:** Many women with PCOS conceive successfully with the right management and treatment.

Insulin Resistance and PCOS

Insulin resistance plays a significant role in PCOS. When your body's cells resist insulin, your pancreas compensates by producing more, leading to higher insulin levels in your blood. This excess insulin can increase androgen production, exacerbating PCOS symptoms like hair growth and acne.

How Insulin Resistance Affects PCOS

- **Weight Gain:** Insulin resistance makes it harder to lose weight, creating a vicious cycle.
- **Hormonal Imbalance:** Excess insulin stimulates androgen production, disrupting the hormonal balance.
- **Inflammation:** Chronic low-grade inflammation is common in women with PCOS and insulin resistance.

The Insulin Resistance Diet

The insulin resistance diet focuses on foods that help maintain stable blood sugar levels. This means prioritizing complex carbohydrates, lean proteins, healthy fats, and plenty of fiber.

Principles of the Diet

- **Complex Carbs:** Opt for whole grains like quinoa, brown rice, and oats over refined grains.
- **Lean Proteins:** Include sources like chicken, fish, tofu, and legumes.
- **Healthy Fats:** Avocados, nuts, seeds, and olive oil are great choices.

- **Fiber-Rich Foods:** Vegetables, fruits, and whole grains help keep you full and manage blood sugar.

Benefits of Following This Diet for PCOS

- **Weight Management:** Helps in maintaining a healthy weight, reducing PCOS symptoms.
- **Improved Insulin Sensitivity:** Stabilizes blood sugar levels and reduces insulin spikes.
- **Hormonal Balance:** Supports overall hormonal health, reducing symptoms like acne and excess hair growth.

Meal Prep Basics

Benefits of Meal Prep for PCOS Management

Managing PCOS can feel like a full-time job, but meal prepping can make it much more manageable. Here are some benefits of meal prepping specifically for PCOS management:

- **Time-Saving Strategies:** By dedicating a few hours each week to meal prep, you save time on daily cooking and cleaning. This efficiency can help you stick to your dietary goals even on the busiest days.
- **Reducing Stress:** Having ready-to-eat, nutritious meals reduces the daily stress of deciding what to eat. This is particularly important for managing cortisol levels, which can impact PCOS symptoms.
- **Improving Adherence to the Diet:** With meals prepared and portioned out, it's easier to stick to your insulin resistance diet and avoid the temptation of unhealthy, quick fixes.

Essential Meal Prep Tools and Ingredients

Kitchen Gadgets and Tools for Efficient Meal Prep:

- **Food Processor:** Perfect for chopping, slicing, and dicing vegetables quickly.

- **Slow Cooker or Instant Pot:** Great for making large batches of soups, stews, and proteins with minimal effort.
- **Mason Jars:** Ideal for storing salads, overnight oats, and smoothies.
- **Glass Storage Containers:** Keep your prepped meals fresh and easy to reheat.
- **Measuring Cups and Spoons:** Essential for accurate portioning.

Staple Ingredients for the Insulin Resistance Diet:

- **Complex Carbs:** Quinoa, brown rice, sweet potatoes, oats, whole grain pasta.
- **Lean Proteins:** Chicken breast, turkey, tofu, tempeh, lentils, beans.
- **Healthy Fats:** Avocados, olive oil, nuts, seeds, fatty fish like salmon.
- **Fiber-Rich Foods:** Leafy greens, broccoli, Brussels sprouts, berries, apples.
- **Spices and Herbs:** Cinnamon, turmeric, garlic, basil, rosemary.

Meal Prep Tips and Tricks

Planning and Organizing Meals:

- **Create a Weekly Menu:** Plan your meals for the week, including breakfast, lunch, dinner, and snacks.
- **Make a Shopping List:** Based on your menu, write down all the ingredients you need to buy.
- **Batch Cooking:** Prepare large quantities of food that can be portioned out and stored for the week.
- **Label and Date:** Clearly label and date your prepped meals to keep track of freshness.

Batch Cooking and Storing Meals:

- **Cook Once, Eat Multiple Times:** Focus on recipes that yield multiple servings. For example, cook a large pot of quinoa or a batch of grilled chicken to use in various meals.
- **Proper Storage:** Use airtight containers to store prepped food in the refrigerator or freezer. Glass containers are preferred for reheating.
- **Freezing Portions:** Freeze portions of meals that you won't consume within a few days. This prevents waste and ensures you have healthy options available.

4

Breakfast Recipes

Importance of a Healthy Breakfast

Starting your day with a healthy breakfast can stabilize your blood sugar levels, which is crucial for managing insulin resistance. A balanced breakfast should include complex carbs, protein, and healthy fats to keep you full and energized throughout the morning.

Easy and Delicious Breakfast Ideas

- **Smoothie Bowls**
- **Overnight Oats**
- **Egg Muffins**

Green Smoothie Bowl

Ingredients:

- 1 cup spinach
- 1 frozen banana
- 1/2 avocado
- 1/2 cup almond milk
- 1 tbsp chia seeds
- 1 tbsp almond butter

- Toppings: Fresh berries, granola, coconut flakes

Instructions:

1. Blend spinach, frozen banana, avocado, almond milk, chia seeds, and almond butter until smooth.
2. Pour into a bowl and top with fresh berries, granola, and coconut flakes.

Nutritional Information (per serving):

- Calories: 350
- Protein: 8g
- Carbs: 45g
- Fat: 17g

Cinnamon Apple Overnight Oats

Ingredients:

- 1/2 cup rolled oats
- 1/2 cup unsweetened almond milk
- 1/4 cup Greek yogurt
- 1 apple, diced
- 1 tsp cinnamon
- 1 tsp honey
- 1 tbsp chia seeds

Instructions:

1. In a mason jar, combine oats, almond milk, Greek yogurt, diced apple, cinnamon, honey, and chia seeds.
2. Stir well, cover, and refrigerate overnight.

3. In the morning, stir again and enjoy.

Nutritional Information (per serving):

- Calories: 250
- Protein: 10g
- Carbs: 45g
- Fat: 5g

Veggie-Packed Egg Muffins

Ingredients:

- 6 large eggs
- 1/4 cup milk
- 1/2 cup diced bell peppers
- 1/2 cup spinach, chopped
- 1/4 cup feta cheese
- Salt and pepper to taste

Instructions:

1. Preheat the oven to 350°F (175°C). Grease a muffin tin or line with silicone cups.
2. In a bowl, whisk together eggs and milk. Add bell peppers, spinach, feta cheese, salt, and pepper.
3. Pour the mixture evenly into the muffin tin.
4. Bake for 20-25 minutes or until the eggs are set.
5. Allow to cool before removing from the tin.

Nutritional Information (per serving - 2 muffins):

- Calories: 180

- Protein: 14g
- Carbs: 4g
- Fat: 12g

Avocado Toast with a Twist

Ingredients:

- 2 slices whole grain bread
- 1 ripe avocado
- 1/2 lemon, juiced
- 1/4 tsp chili flakes
- Salt and pepper to taste
- Optional: Poached egg, cherry tomatoes, arugula

Instructions:

1. Toast the whole grain bread slices until golden brown.
2. In a bowl, mash the avocado with lemon juice, chili flakes, salt, and pepper.
3. Spread the avocado mixture evenly on the toast.
4. Top with optional poached egg, cherry tomatoes, and arugula if desired.

Nutritional Information (per serving):

- Calories: 300
- Protein: 8g
- Carbs: 32g
- Fat: 18g

Chia Seed Pudding with Berries

Ingredients:

- 1/4 cup chia seeds
- 1 cup unsweetened almond milk
- 1 tsp vanilla extract
- 1 tbsp maple syrup
- Fresh berries for topping

Instructions:

1. In a bowl, mix chia seeds, almond milk, vanilla extract, and maple syrup.
2. Stir well and refrigerate overnight.
3. In the morning, stir the pudding and top with fresh berries.

Nutritional Information (per serving):

- Calories: 200
- Protein: 6g
- Carbs: 25g
- Fat: 10g

Spinach and Feta Breakfast Wrap

Ingredients:

- 1 whole wheat tortilla
- 1/2 cup spinach, chopped
- 1/4 cup feta cheese, crumbled
- 2 large eggs
- 1 tbsp olive oil

- Salt and pepper to taste

Instructions:

1. Heat olive oil in a pan over medium heat.
2. Add spinach and cook until wilted.
3. In a bowl, whisk the eggs with salt and pepper, then pour into the pan with the spinach.
4. Cook until the eggs are set, then remove from heat and add feta cheese.
5. Place the egg mixture in the center of the tortilla and wrap it up.

Nutritional Information (per serving):

- Calories: 350
- Protein: 18g
- Carbs: 25g
- Fat: 20g

Greek Yogurt Parfait

Ingredients:

- 1 cup Greek yogurt
- 1/2 cup granola
- 1/2 cup mixed berries
- 1 tbsp honey

Instructions:

1. Layer Greek yogurt, granola, and mixed berries in a bowl or jar.
2. Drizzle with honey and enjoy.

Nutritional Information (per serving):

- Calories: 350
- Protein: 15g
- Carbs: 50g
- Fat: 10g

Almond Flour Pancakes

Ingredients:

- 1 cup almond flour
- 2 large eggs
- 1/4 cup almond milk
- 1 tsp baking powder
- 1 tsp vanilla extract
- 1 tbsp maple syrup
- Olive oil for cooking

Instructions:

1. In a bowl, mix almond flour, eggs, almond milk, baking powder, vanilla extract, and maple syrup until smooth.
2. Heat olive oil in a pan over medium heat.
3. Pour 1/4 cup of batter for each pancake into the pan.
4. Cook until bubbles form on the surface, then flip and cook until golden brown.

Nutritional Information (per serving - 3 pancakes):

- Calories: 300
- Protein: 12g
- Carbs: 12g

- Fat: 24g

Tofu Scramble

Ingredients:

- 1 block firm tofu, crumbled
- 1/2 onion, diced
- 1/2 bell pepper, diced
- 1 cup spinach, chopped
- 1 tbsp olive oil
- 1/2 tsp turmeric
- Salt and pepper to taste

Instructions:

1. Heat olive oil in a pan over medium heat.
2. Add onion and bell pepper, cook until softened.
3. Add crumbled tofu, turmeric, salt, and pepper, and cook until heated through.
4. Add spinach and cook until wilted.

Nutritional Information (per serving):

- Calories: 200
- Protein: 18g
- Carbs: 8g
- Fat: 12g

Quinoa Breakfast Bowl

Ingredients:

- 1/2 cup cooked quinoa
- 1/4 avocado, sliced
- 1 poached egg
- 1 tbsp salsa
- 1 tbsp chopped cilantro

Instructions:

1. In a bowl, combine cooked quinoa, avocado slices, and poached egg.
2. Top with salsa and chopped cilantro.

Nutritional Information (per serving):

- Calories: 250
- Protein: 10g
- Carbs: 28g
- Fat: 12g

Breakfast Burrito

Ingredients:

- 1 whole wheat tortilla
- 2 large eggs
- 1/4 cup black beans
- 1/4 cup diced tomatoes
- 1/4 avocado, sliced
- 1 tbsp shredded cheese
- Salsa for serving

Instructions:

1. In a pan, scramble the eggs and cook until set.
2. Warm the tortilla and layer with eggs, black beans, diced tomatoes, avocado slices, and shredded cheese.
3. Roll up the tortilla and serve with salsa.

Nutritional Information (per serving):

- Calories: 350
- Protein: 18g
- Carbs: 35g
- Fat: 18g

Protein-Packed Smoothie

Ingredients:

- 1 cup unsweetened almond milk
- 1 scoop protein powder (vanilla or chocolate)
- 1 frozen banana
- 1 tbsp almond butter
- 1 tbsp chia seeds

Instructions:

1. Blend all ingredients until smooth.
2. Pour into a glass and enjoy.

Nutritional Information (per serving):

- Calories: 300
- Protein: 20g
- Carbs: 30g
- Fat: 12g

Sweet Potato Hash

Ingredients:

- 1 medium sweet potato, diced
- 1/2 onion, diced
- 1/2 bell pepper, diced
- 1 tbsp olive oil
- 1/2 tsp paprika
- Salt and pepper to taste
- 2 large eggs

Instructions:

1. Heat olive oil in a pan over medium heat.
2. Add sweet potato, onion, bell pepper, paprika, salt, and pepper.
3. Cook until sweet potatoes are tender and crispy.
4. In a separate pan, fry or scramble the eggs.
5. Serve eggs over sweet potato hash.

Nutritional Information (per serving):

- Calories: 300
- Protein: 10g
- Carbs: 35g
- Fat: 15g

Mushroom Omelette

Ingredients:

- 2 large eggs
- 1/2 cup mushrooms, sliced

- 1/4 cup spinach, chopped
- 1 tbsp olive oil
- Salt and pepper to taste

Instructions:

1. Heat olive oil in a pan over medium heat.
2. Add mushrooms and cook until soft.
3. Add spinach and cook until wilted.
4. In a bowl, whisk eggs with salt and pepper.
5. Pour eggs into the pan with vegetables and cook until set.
6. Fold omelette in half and serve.

Nutritional Information (per serving):

- Calories: 200
- Protein: 12g
- Carbs: 4g
- Fat: 16g

Keto Breakfast Sandwich

Ingredients:

- 2 large eggs
- 2 slices of turkey bacon
- 1 slice of cheddar cheese
- 1/4 avocado, sliced
- Salt and pepper to taste

Instructions:

1. Cook turkey bacon in a pan until crispy.

2. In a separate pan, cook eggs to your liking (fried or scrambled).

3. Layer eggs, turkey bacon, cheese, and avocado slices on a plate.

4. Season with salt and pepper and serve.

Nutritional Information (per serving):

- Calories: 300
- Protein: 20g
- Carbs: 6g
- Fat: 22g

5

Lunch Recipes

Balanced Lunch Options for Insulin Control

A balanced lunch can help maintain stable blood sugar levels throughout the day, which is crucial for managing insulin resistance and PCOS. Focus on incorporating lean proteins, healthy fats, and complex carbohydrates to create satisfying and nutritious meals.

Quick and Easy Lunch Ideas

- **Salads**
- **Wraps**
- **Grain Bowls**

Mediterranean Chickpea Salad

Ingredients:

- 1 can chickpeas, drained and rinsed
- 1 cup cherry tomatoes, halved
- 1 cucumber, diced
- 1/4 cup red onion, thinly sliced
- 1/4 cup Kalamata olives, pitted and halved
- 1/4 cup feta cheese, crumbled
- 2 tbsp olive oil
- 1 tbsp red wine vinegar

- 1 tsp dried oregano
- Salt and pepper to taste

Instructions:

1. In a large bowl, combine chickpeas, cherry tomatoes, cucumber, red onion, olives, and feta cheese.
2. In a small bowl, whisk together olive oil, red wine vinegar, oregano, salt, and pepper.
3. Pour the dressing over the salad and toss to combine.

Nutritional Information (per serving):

- Calories: 300
- Protein: 10g
- Carbs: 30g
- Fat: 16g

Grilled Chicken Caesar Wrap

Ingredients:

- 1 whole wheat tortilla
- 1 grilled chicken breast, sliced
- 1 cup romaine lettuce, chopped
- 1/4 cup grated Parmesan cheese
- 2 tbsp Caesar dressing
- 1/4 cup cherry tomatoes, halved

Instructions:

1. Lay the whole wheat tortilla flat and layer with romaine lettuce, grilled chicken slices, Parmesan cheese, cherry tomatoes, and Caesar dressing.
2. Roll up the tortilla tightly and slice in half.

Nutritional Information (per serving):

- Calories: 350
- Protein: 30g
- Carbs: 30g
- Fat: 14g

Quinoa and Black Bean Salad

Ingredients:

- 1 cup cooked quinoa
- 1 can black beans, drained and rinsed
- 1 red bell pepper, diced
- 1/4 cup red onion, diced
- 1/2 cup corn kernels
- 1/4 cup cilantro, chopped
- 2 tbsp lime juice
- 1 tbsp olive oil
- Salt and pepper to taste

Instructions:

1. In a large bowl, combine cooked quinoa, black beans, red bell pepper, red onion, corn, and cilantro.
2. In a small bowl, whisk together lime juice, olive oil, salt, and pepper.
3. Pour the dressing over the salad and toss to combine.

Nutritional Information (per serving):

- Calories: 350
- Protein: 12g
- Carbs: 50g
- Fat: 10g

Turkey Avocado Club

Ingredients:

- 2 slices whole grain bread
- 4 slices turkey breast
- 1/4 avocado, sliced
- 2 slices tomato
- 1 leaf lettuce
- 1 tbsp mustard

Instructions:

1. Toast the whole grain bread slices until golden brown.
2. Spread mustard on one slice of bread.
3. Layer with turkey breast, avocado slices, tomato, and lettuce.
4. Top with the other slice of bread and cut in half.

Nutritional Information (per serving):

- Calories: 350
- Protein: 20g
- Carbs: 40g
- Fat: 12g

Thai Peanut Noodle Bowl

Ingredients:

- 4 oz whole wheat noodles
- 1/2 cup shredded carrots
- 1/2 cup bell peppers, sliced
- 1/4 cup edamame
- 1/4 cup green onions, sliced
- 1/4 cup chopped peanuts
- 2 tbsp peanut butter
- 1 tbsp soy sauce
- 1 tbsp lime juice
- 1 tsp honey
- 1/4 tsp red pepper flakes
- 1 tbsp water

Instructions:

1. Cook whole wheat noodles according to package instructions and drain.
2. In a small bowl, whisk together peanut butter, soy sauce, lime juice, honey, red pepper flakes, and water until smooth.
3. In a large bowl, combine cooked noodles, shredded carrots, bell peppers, edamame, and green onions.
4. Pour the peanut dressing over the noodle mixture and toss to combine.
5. Top with chopped peanuts before serving.

Nutritional Information (per serving):

- Calories: 400
- Protein: 15g

- Carbs: 50g
- Fat: 18g

Greek Salad with Lemon Dressing

Ingredients:

- 2 cups mixed greens
- 1/2 cup cherry tomatoes, halved
- 1/2 cucumber, sliced
- 1/4 cup red onion, thinly sliced
- 1/4 cup Kalamata olives, pitted and halved
- 1/4 cup feta cheese, crumbled
- 2 tbsp olive oil
- 1 tbsp lemon juice
- 1 tsp dried oregano
- Salt and pepper to taste

Instructions:

1. In a large bowl, combine mixed greens, cherry tomatoes, cucumber, red onion, olives, and feta cheese.
2. In a small bowl, whisk together olive oil, lemon juice, oregano, salt, and pepper.
3. Pour the dressing over the salad and toss to combine.

Nutritional Information (per serving):

- Calories: 250
- Protein: 6g
- Carbs: 12g
- Fat: 20g

Lentil Soup

Ingredients:

- 1 cup lentils, rinsed
- 1 onion, diced
- 2 carrots, diced
- 2 celery stalks, diced
- 3 garlic cloves, minced
- 1 can diced tomatoes
- 4 cups vegetable broth
- 1 tsp cumin
- 1 tsp paprika
- 1 bay leaf
- Salt and pepper to taste
- 2 tbsp olive oil

Instructions:

1. Heat olive oil in a large pot over medium heat. Add onion, carrots, and celery, and cook until softened.
2. Add garlic and cook for another minute.
3. Add lentils, diced tomatoes, vegetable broth, cumin, paprika, bay leaf, salt, and pepper. Bring to a boil.
4. Reduce heat and simmer for 30-35 minutes, or until lentils are tender.
5. Remove bay leaf before serving.

Nutritional Information (per serving):

- Calories: 300
- Protein: 15g
- Carbs: 40g

- Fat: 8g

Shrimp and Avocado Salad

Ingredients:

- 1/2 lb cooked shrimp, peeled and deveined
- 1 avocado, diced
- 1 cup cherry tomatoes, halved
- 1/2 cucumber, diced
- 1/4 cup red onion, thinly sliced
- 2 tbsp olive oil
- 1 tbsp lime juice
- Salt and pepper to taste

Instructions:

1. In a large bowl, combine shrimp, avocado, cherry tomatoes, cucumber, and red onion.
2. In a small bowl, whisk together olive oil, lime juice, salt, and pepper.
3. Pour the dressing over the salad and toss to combine.

Nutritional Information (per serving):

- Calories: 300
- Protein: 20g
- Carbs: 12g
- Fat: 20g

Vegan Buddha Bowl

Ingredients:

- 1/2 cup cooked quinoa
- 1/2 cup roasted sweet potatoes
- 1/4 cup chickpeas, roasted
- 1/2 avocado, sliced
- 1/2 cup spinach
- 1 tbsp tahini
- 1 tbsp lemon juice
- Salt and pepper to taste

Instructions:

1. In a bowl, layer cooked quinoa, roasted sweet potatoes, roasted chickpeas, avocado slices, and spinach.
2. In a small bowl, mix tahini, lemon juice, salt, and pepper to make the dressing.
3. Drizzle the tahini dressing over the bowl before serving.

Nutritional Information (per serving):

- Calories: 350
- Protein: 12g
- Carbs: 45g
- Fat: 16g

Spinach and Quinoa Stuffed Peppers

Ingredients:

- 4 bell peppers, tops cut off and seeds removed
- 1 cup cooked quinoa
- 2 cups spinach, chopped
- 1/2 cup feta cheese, crumbled
- 1/4 cup sun-dried tomatoes, chopped

- 1 onion, diced
- 2 garlic cloves, minced
- 2 tbsp olive oil
- Salt and pepper to taste

Instructions:

1. Preheat oven to 375°F (190°C).
2. Heat olive oil in a pan over medium heat. Add onion and garlic, and cook until softened.
3. Add spinach and cook until wilted.
4. In a bowl, mix cooked quinoa, spinach mixture, feta cheese, sun-dried tomatoes, salt, and pepper.
5. Stuff the bell peppers with the quinoa mixture and place them in a baking dish.
6. Bake for 25-30 minutes until peppers are tender.

Nutritional Information (per serving):

- Calories: 300
- Protein: 10g
- Carbs: 40g
- Fat: 12g

Chicken and Veggie Stir-Fry

Ingredients:

- 1 lb chicken breast, thinly sliced
- 1 red bell pepper, sliced
- 1 broccoli crown, cut into florets
- 1 carrot, julienned
- 2 garlic cloves, minced

- 2 tbsp soy sauce
- 1 tbsp olive oil
- 1 tsp sesame oil
- 1 tsp ginger, grated

Instructions:

1. Heat olive oil in a pan over medium-high heat.
2. Add chicken slices and cook until browned.
3. Add garlic and ginger, and cook for another minute.
4. Add bell pepper, broccoli, and carrot, and stir-fry until vegetables are tender.
5. Add soy sauce and sesame oil, and toss to combine.

Nutritional Information (per serving):

- Calories: 350
- Protein: 30g
- Carbs: 15g
- Fat: 18g

Tuna Salad Lettuce Wraps

Ingredients:

- 1 can tuna, drained
- 1/4 cup Greek yogurt
- 1/4 cup celery, diced
- 1/4 cup red onion, diced
- 1 tbsp lemon juice
- Salt and pepper to taste
- Romaine lettuce leaves

Instructions:

1. In a bowl, mix tuna, Greek yogurt, celery, red onion, lemon juice, salt, and pepper.
2. Spoon the tuna mixture onto romaine lettuce leaves and wrap them up.

Nutritional Information (per serving):

- Calories: 200
- Protein: 20g
- Carbs: 8g
- Fat: 8g

Falafel Bowl

Ingredients:

- 4 falafel patties, cooked
- 1 cup mixed greens
- 1/2 cup cherry tomatoes, halved
- 1/4 cup cucumber, diced
- 1/4 cup red onion, sliced
- 2 tbsp hummus
- 1 tbsp lemon juice
- 1 tbsp olive oil
- Salt and pepper to taste

Instructions:

1. In a bowl, layer mixed greens, cherry tomatoes, cucumber, red onion, and falafel patties.

2. In a small bowl, whisk together hummus, lemon juice, olive oil, salt, and pepper.
3. Drizzle the hummus dressing over the bowl before serving.

Nutritional Information (per serving):

- Calories: 350
- Protein: 10g
- Carbs: 45g
- Fat: 14g

Zucchini Noodles with Pesto

Ingredients:

- 2 zucchinis, spiralized
- 1/4 cup basil pesto
- 1/4 cup cherry tomatoes, halved
- 2 tbsp pine nuts, toasted
- 1 tbsp olive oil
- Salt and pepper to taste

Instructions:

1. Heat olive oil in a pan over medium heat.
2. Add zucchini noodles and cook for 2-3 minutes until tender.
3. Remove from heat and toss with basil pesto, cherry tomatoes, pine nuts, salt, and pepper.

Nutritional Information (per serving):

- Calories: 200
- Protein: 6g

- Carbs: 12g
- Fat: 16g

Spaghetti Squash Pad Thai

Ingredients:

- 1 spaghetti squash, cooked and shredded
- 1/2 lb shrimp, peeled and deveined
- 1/2 cup carrots, julienned
- 1/4 cup green onions, sliced
- 1/4 cup peanuts, chopped
- 2 tbsp soy sauce
- 1 tbsp lime juice
- 1 tbsp olive oil
- 1 tsp honey
- 1/4 tsp red pepper flakes

Instructions:

1. Heat olive oil in a pan over medium heat.
2. Add shrimp and cook until pink and opaque.
3. Add carrots and green onions, and cook for another minute.
4. In a small bowl, whisk together soy sauce, lime juice, honey, and red pepper flakes.
5. Add cooked spaghetti squash to the pan and pour the sauce over it. Toss to combine.
6. Top with chopped peanuts before serving.

Nutritional Information (per serving):

- Calories: 300
- Protein: 20g

- Carbs: 25g
- Fat: 12g

Cauliflower Rice Bowl

Ingredients:

- 1 cup cauliflower rice
- 1/2 cup black beans, drained and rinsed
- 1/2 avocado, diced
- 1/2 cup corn kernels
- 1/4 cup salsa
- 1 tbsp lime juice
- 1 tbsp cilantro, chopped
- Salt and pepper to taste

Instructions:

1. Cook cauliflower rice according to package instructions.
2. In a bowl, layer cauliflower rice, black beans, avocado, corn, and salsa.
3. Drizzle with lime juice and top with chopped cilantro, salt, and pepper.

Nutritional Information (per serving):

- Calories: 250
- Protein: 10g
- Carbs: 30g
- Fat: 12g

Roasted Veggie Wrap

Ingredients:

- 1 whole wheat tortilla
- 1/2 cup roasted vegetables (bell peppers, zucchini, eggplant)
- 1/4 cup hummus
- 1/4 cup spinach
- 1 tbsp feta cheese, crumbled

Instructions:

1. Spread hummus on the whole wheat tortilla.
2. Layer with roasted vegetables, spinach, and feta cheese.
3. Roll up the tortilla and slice in half.

Nutritional Information (per serving):

- Calories: 300
- Protein: 10g
- Carbs: 40g
- Fat: 12g

Salmon Salad with Dill Dressing

Ingredients:

- 1 can salmon, drained
- 1/4 cup Greek yogurt
- 1 tbsp dill, chopped
- 1 tbsp lemon juice
- 1/4 cup cucumber, diced
- Salt and pepper to taste

- Romaine lettuce leaves

Instructions:

1. In a bowl, mix salmon, Greek yogurt, dill, lemon juice, cucumber, salt, and pepper.
2. Spoon the salmon mixture onto romaine lettuce leaves and wrap them up.

Nutritional Information (per serving):

- Calories: 250
- Protein: 20g
- Carbs: 8g
- Fat: 12g

Edamame and Brown Rice Bowl

Ingredients:

- 1 cup cooked brown rice
- 1/2 cup edamame, shelled
- 1/4 cup carrots, julienned
- 1/4 cup red cabbage, shredded
- 1 tbsp sesame seeds
- 2 tbsp soy sauce
- 1 tbsp rice vinegar
- 1 tbsp sesame oil

Instructions:

1. In a bowl, layer cooked brown rice, edamame, carrots, and red cabbage.

2. In a small bowl, whisk together soy sauce, rice vinegar, and sesame oil.
3. Pour the dressing over the bowl and top with sesame seeds.

Nutritional Information (per serving):

- Calories: 350
- Protein: 12g
- Carbs: 50g
- Fat: 12g

BBQ Chicken Salad

Ingredients:

- 1 grilled chicken breast, sliced
- 2 cups mixed greens
- 1/4 cup corn kernels
- 1/4 cup black beans, drained and rinsed
- 1/4 cup cherry tomatoes, halved
- 2 tbsp BBQ sauce
- 1 tbsp ranch dressing

Instructions:

1. In a bowl, layer mixed greens, grilled chicken slices, corn, black beans, and cherry tomatoes.
2. Drizzle with BBQ sauce and ranch dressing before serving.

Nutritional Information (per serving):

- Calories: 300
- Protein: 25g

- Carbs: 30g
- Fat: 10g

6

Dinner Recipes

Nutritious and Satisfying Dinner Choices

Dinner is an important meal for maintaining insulin control over-night. Focus on combining lean proteins, healthy fats, and complex carbohydrates to create satisfying and nutritious meals.

Simple and Flavorful Dinner Ideas

- **One-Pot Meals**
- **Sheet Pan Dinners**
- **Stir-Fries**

Baked Lemon Herb Chicken

Ingredients:

- 4 boneless, skinless chicken breasts
- 1/4 cup olive oil
- 2 tbsp lemon juice
- 2 garlic cloves, minced
- 1 tbsp dried oregano
- 1 tsp dried thyme
- Salt and pepper to taste
- Lemon slices for garnish

Instructions:

1. Preheat oven to 375°F (190°C).
2. In a small bowl, mix olive oil, lemon juice, garlic, oregano, thyme, salt, and pepper.
3. Place chicken breasts in a baking dish and pour the olive oil mixture over them, turning to coat.
4. Bake for 25-30 minutes or until the chicken is cooked through.
5. Garnish with lemon slices before serving.

Nutritional Information (per serving):

- Calories: 250
- Protein: 30g
- Carbs: 2g
- Fat: 14g

Garlic Shrimp Stir-Fry

Ingredients:

- 1 lb shrimp, peeled and deveined
- 1 red bell pepper, sliced
- 1 yellow bell pepper, sliced
- 1 cup snap peas
- 3 garlic cloves, minced
- 2 tbsp soy sauce
- 1 tbsp olive oil
- 1 tsp sesame oil
- 1 tsp grated ginger

Instructions:

1. Heat olive oil in a large pan over medium-high heat.
2. Add garlic and ginger, and cook for 1 minute.
3. Add shrimp and cook until pink, then remove from the pan.
4. Add bell peppers and snap peas to the pan, and stir-fry until tender.
5. Return shrimp to the pan and add soy sauce and sesame oil. Toss to combine.

Nutritional Information (per serving):

- Calories: 200
- Protein: 25g
- Carbs: 10g
- Fat: 8g

Beef and Broccoli

Ingredients:

- 1 lb beef sirloin, thinly sliced
- 2 cups broccoli florets
- 1/2 onion, sliced
- 2 garlic cloves, minced
- 2 tbsp soy sauce
- 1 tbsp oyster sauce
- 1 tbsp olive oil
- 1 tsp cornstarch
- 1/2 cup beef broth

Instructions:

1. In a small bowl, mix soy sauce, oyster sauce, cornstarch, and beef broth.

2. Heat olive oil in a pan over medium-high heat.
3. Add garlic and onion, and cook until fragrant.
4. Add beef slices and cook until browned.
5. Add broccoli florets and the sauce mixture. Cook until the broccoli is tender and the sauce has thickened.

Nutritional Information (per serving):

- Calories: 300
- Protein: 25g
- Carbs: 12g
- Fat: 16g

Spaghetti Squash Bolognese

Ingredients:

- 1 spaghetti squash
- 1 lb ground turkey
- 1 onion, diced
- 2 garlic cloves, minced
- 1 can crushed tomatoes
- 1 tsp dried basil
- 1 tsp dried oregano
- 1/2 tsp salt
- 1/4 tsp black pepper
- 2 tbsp olive oil

Instructions:

1. Preheat oven to 375°F (190°C).

2. Cut the spaghetti squash in half, remove seeds, and brush with olive oil. Place cut-side down on a baking sheet and bake for 40-45 minutes.

3. While the squash is baking, heat olive oil in a pan over medium heat. Add onion and garlic, and cook until softened.

4. Add ground turkey and cook until browned.

5. Stir in crushed tomatoes, basil, oregano, salt, and pepper. Simmer for 20 minutes.

6. Use a fork to scrape out the spaghetti squash strands and serve topped with the turkey Bolognese sauce.

Nutritional Information (per serving):

- Calories: 350
- Protein: 25g
- Carbs: 30g
- Fat: 14g

Veggie-Packed Chili

Ingredients:

- 1 can black beans, drained and rinsed
- 1 can kidney beans, drained and rinsed
- 1 can diced tomatoes
- 1 onion, diced
- 1 red bell pepper, diced
- 1 zucchini, diced
- 2 garlic cloves, minced
- 1 tbsp chili powder
- 1 tsp cumin
- 1 tsp paprika
- 2 tbsp olive oil

- Salt and pepper to taste

Instructions:

1. Heat olive oil in a large pot over medium heat. Add onion and garlic, and cook until softened.
2. Add bell pepper and zucchini, and cook for another 5 minutes.
3. Stir in black beans, kidney beans, diced tomatoes, chili powder, cumin, paprika, salt, and pepper.
4. Simmer for 20-25 minutes, stirring occasionally.

Nutritional Information (per serving):

- Calories: 300
- Protein: 15g
- Carbs: 50g
- Fat: 8g

Herb-Crusted Salmon

Ingredients:

- 4 salmon fillets
- 2 tbsp Dijon mustard
- 1/4 cup panko breadcrumbs
- 1/4 cup Parmesan cheese, grated
- 2 tbsp fresh parsley, chopped
- 1 tbsp olive oil
- Salt and pepper to taste

Instructions:

1. Preheat oven to 400°F (200°C).

2. Place salmon fillets on a baking sheet lined with parchment paper. Spread Dijon mustard over each fillet.

3. In a small bowl, mix panko breadcrumbs, Parmesan cheese, parsley, olive oil, salt, and pepper.

4. Press the breadcrumb mixture onto the top of each salmon fillet.

5. Bake for 12-15 minutes or until the salmon is cooked through and the crust is golden brown.

Nutritional Information (per serving):

- Calories: 350
- Protein: 30g
- Carbs: 10g
- Fat: 20g

Chicken and Zucchini Skillet

Ingredients:

- 1 lb chicken breast, cut into cubes
- 2 zucchinis, sliced
- 1 red bell pepper, sliced
- 1 onion, diced
- 3 garlic cloves, minced
- 2 tbsp olive oil
- 1 tsp Italian seasoning
- Salt and pepper to taste

Instructions:

1. Heat olive oil in a large skillet over medium heat. Add onion and garlic, and cook until softened.

2. Add chicken cubes, and cook until browned and cooked through.

3. Add zucchini and bell pepper, and cook until tender.
4. Stir in Italian seasoning, salt, and pepper.

Nutritional Information (per serving):

- Calories: 300
- Protein: 30g
- Carbs: 10g
- Fat: 16g

Vegan Lentil Curry

Ingredients:

- 1 cup lentils, rinsed
- 1 can coconut milk
- 1 can diced tomatoes
- 1 onion, diced
- 2 garlic cloves, minced
- 1 tbsp curry powder
- 1 tsp cumin
- 1 tsp turmeric
- 2 tbsp olive oil
- Salt and pepper to taste

Instructions:

1. Heat olive oil in a large pot over medium heat. Add onion and garlic, and cook until softened.
2. Stir in curry powder, cumin, and turmeric, and cook for another minute.
3. Add lentils, coconut milk, diced tomatoes, salt, and pepper. Bring to a boil.

4. Reduce heat and simmer for 25-30 minutes or until lentils are tender.

Nutritional Information (per serving):

- Calories: 350
- Protein: 12g
- Carbs: 40g
- Fat: 16g

Turkey Meatballs with Zoodles

Ingredients:

- 1 lb ground turkey
- 1/4 cup breadcrumbs
- 1/4 cup Parmesan cheese, grated
- 1 egg
- 2 garlic cloves, minced
- 1 tsp dried basil
- 1 tsp dried oregano
- 2 zucchinis, spiralized
- 1 jar marinara sauce
- 2 tbsp olive oil
- Salt and pepper to taste

Instructions:

1. Preheat oven to 375°F (190°C).
2. In a bowl, mix ground turkey, breadcrumbs, Parmesan cheese, egg, garlic, basil, oregano, salt, and pepper. Form into meatballs.
3. Place meatballs on a baking sheet and bake for 20-25 minutes or until cooked through.

4. While the meatballs are baking, heat olive oil in a pan over medium heat. Add spiralized zucchini and cook for 2-3 minutes until tender.
5. Heat marinara sauce in a separate pot.
6. Serve meatballs over zoodles, topped with marinara sauce.

Nutritional Information (per serving):

- Calories: 350
- Protein: 25g
- Carbs: 20g
- Fat: 18g

Balsamic Glazed Pork Chops

Ingredients:

- 4 boneless pork chops
- 1/4 cup balsamic vinegar
- 2 tbsp honey
- 2 garlic cloves, minced
- 1 tbsp olive oil
- Salt and pepper to taste

Instructions:

1. In a small bowl, mix balsamic vinegar, honey, and garlic.
2. Heat olive oil in a pan over medium-high heat.
3. Season pork chops with salt and pepper, and add to the pan. Cook until browned on both sides.
4. Pour the balsamic mixture over the pork chops and cook for another 5-7 minutes, or until the glaze has thickened and the pork chops are cooked through.

Nutritional Information (per serving):

- Calories: 300
- Protein: 30g
- Carbs: 10g
- Fat: 14g

Thai Green Curry

Ingredients:

- 1 lb chicken breast, sliced
- 1 can coconut milk
- 2 tbsp green curry paste
- 1 cup broccoli florets
- 1 red bell pepper, sliced
- 1 carrot, sliced
- 1 tbsp olive oil
- 1 tbsp fish sauce
- 1 tbsp lime juice

Instructions:

1. Heat olive oil in a large pot over medium heat. Add green curry paste and cook for 1 minute.
2. Add chicken slices and cook until browned.
3. Stir in coconut milk, broccoli, bell pepper, and carrot. Bring to a boil.
4. Reduce heat and simmer for 15 minutes or until vegetables are tender.
5. Stir in fish sauce and lime juice before serving.

Nutritional Information (per serving):

- Calories: 350
- Protein: 25g
- Carbs: 15g
- Fat: 20g

Pesto Chicken Bake

Ingredients:

- 4 boneless, skinless chicken breasts
- 1/2 cup basil pesto
- 1/4 cup cherry tomatoes, halved
- 1/4 cup mozzarella cheese, shredded
- 2 tbsp olive oil
- Salt and pepper to taste

Instructions:

1. Preheat oven to 375°F (190°C).
2. Place chicken breasts in a baking dish and brush with olive oil. Season with salt and pepper.
3. Spread basil pesto over each chicken breast and top with cherry tomatoes and mozzarella cheese.
4. Bake for 25-30 minutes or until the chicken is cooked through and the cheese is melted and bubbly.

Nutritional Information (per serving):

- Calories: 350
- Protein: 30g
- Carbs: 5g
- Fat: 22g

Stuffed Bell Peppers

Ingredients:

- 4 bell peppers, tops cut off and seeds removed
- 1 cup cooked quinoa
- 1/2 lb ground beef
- 1 can diced tomatoes
- 1 onion, diced
- 2 garlic cloves, minced
- 1 tsp cumin
- 1 tsp paprika
- 2 tbsp olive oil
- Salt and pepper to taste

Instructions:

1. Preheat oven to 375°F (190°C).
2. Heat olive oil in a pan over medium heat. Add onion and garlic, and cook until softened.
3. Add ground beef and cook until browned.
4. Stir in cooked quinoa, diced tomatoes, cumin, paprika, salt, and pepper.
5. Stuff the bell peppers with the quinoa mixture and place them in a baking dish.
6. Bake for 25-30 minutes or until the peppers are tender.

Nutritional Information (per serving):

- Calories: 350
- Protein: 20g
- Carbs: 35g
- Fat: 16g

BBQ Cauliflower Tacos

Ingredients:

- 1 head cauliflower, cut into florets
- 1/4 cup BBQ sauce
- 1 tbsp olive oil
- 8 small corn tortillas
- 1/2 cup red cabbage, shredded
- 1/4 cup cilantro, chopped
- 1 lime, cut into wedges
- Salt and pepper to taste

Instructions:

1. Preheat oven to 400°F (200°C).
2. Toss cauliflower florets with olive oil, salt, and pepper, and spread them on a baking sheet. Roast for 20-25 minutes until tender and slightly crispy.
3. Toss roasted cauliflower with BBQ sauce.
4. Warm corn tortillas and fill with BBQ cauliflower, red cabbage, and cilantro. Serve with lime wedges.

Nutritional Information (per serving):

- Calories: 200
- Protein: 4g
- Carbs: 30g
- Fat: 8g

Moroccan Chickpea Stew

Ingredients:

- 2 cans chickpeas, drained and rinsed
- 1 can diced tomatoes
- 1 onion, diced
- 2 garlic cloves, minced
- 1 carrot, diced
- 1 sweet potato, diced
- 1 tsp cumin
- 1 tsp coriander
- 1 tsp paprika
- 1/2 tsp cinnamon
- 2 tbsp olive oil
- 4 cups vegetable broth
- Salt and pepper to taste

Instructions:

1. Heat olive oil in a large pot over medium heat. Add onion and garlic, and cook until softened.
2. Add carrot and sweet potato, and cook for another 5 minutes.
3. Stir in chickpeas, diced tomatoes, vegetable broth, cumin, coriander, paprika, cinnamon, salt, and pepper.
4. Bring to a boil, then reduce heat and simmer for 30-35 minutes or until vegetables are tender.

Nutritional Information (per serving):

- Calories: 300
- Protein: 10g
- Carbs: 50g
- Fat: 8g

Lemon Garlic Tilapia

Ingredients:

- 4 tilapia fillets
- 2 tbsp olive oil
- 2 tbsp lemon juice
- 2 garlic cloves, minced
- 1 tsp dried parsley
- Salt and pepper to taste
- Lemon wedges for serving

Instructions:

1. Preheat oven to 375°F (190°C).
2. Place tilapia fillets in a baking dish. In a small bowl, mix olive oil, lemon juice, garlic, parsley, salt, and pepper.
3. Pour the mixture over the tilapia fillets.
4. Bake for 15-20 minutes or until the fish is cooked through.
5. Serve with lemon wedges.

Nutritional Information (per serving):

- Calories: 250
- Protein: 30g
- Carbs: 2g
- Fat: 14g

Chicken Fajita Bowl

Ingredients:

- 1 lb chicken breast, sliced

- 1 red bell pepper, sliced
- 1 yellow bell pepper, sliced
- 1 onion, sliced
- 2 garlic cloves, minced
- 2 tbsp olive oil
- 1 tsp chili powder
- 1 tsp cumin
- 1 tsp paprika
- 1 cup cooked brown rice
- 1/4 cup salsa
- 1/4 cup guacamole
- Salt and pepper to taste

Instructions:

1. Heat olive oil in a large pan over medium-high heat.
2. Add garlic, chicken slices, chili powder, cumin, paprika, salt, and pepper. Cook until the chicken is browned and cooked through.
3. Add bell peppers and onion, and cook until tender.
4. Serve the chicken and vegetable mixture over cooked brown rice. Top with salsa and guacamole.

Nutritional Information (per serving):

- Calories: 350
- Protein: 30g
- Carbs: 35g
- Fat: 14g

Mediterranean Lamb Stew

Ingredients:

- 1 lb lamb shoulder, cut into cubes
- 1 can diced tomatoes
- 1 onion, diced
- 2 garlic cloves, minced
- 1 cup carrots, sliced
- 1 cup potatoes, diced
- 1 tsp cumin
- 1 tsp paprika
- 1/2 tsp cinnamon
- 2 tbsp olive oil
- 4 cups beef broth
- Salt and pepper to taste

Instructions:

1. Heat olive oil in a large pot over medium heat. Add lamb and brown on all sides.
2. Add onion and garlic, and cook until softened.
3. Stir in diced tomatoes, beef broth, carrots, potatoes, cumin, paprika, cinnamon, salt, and pepper.
4. Bring to a boil, then reduce heat and simmer for 1-1.5 hours or until the lamb is tender.

Nutritional Information (per serving):

- Calories: 400
- Protein: 25g
- Carbs: 35g
- Fat: 18g

Spinach and Ricotta Stuffed Mushrooms

Ingredients:

- 12 large mushroom caps
- 1 cup ricotta cheese
- 1 cup spinach, chopped
- 1/4 cup Parmesan cheese, grated
- 2 garlic cloves, minced
- 1 tbsp olive oil
- Salt and pepper to taste

Instructions:

1. Preheat oven to 375°F (190°C).
2. In a bowl, mix ricotta cheese, chopped spinach, Parmesan cheese, garlic, salt, and pepper.
3. Stuff each mushroom cap with the ricotta mixture.
4. Place stuffed mushrooms on a baking sheet and bake for 20-25 minutes or until the mushrooms are tender.

Nutritional Information (per serving):

- Calories: 200
- Protein: 10g
- Carbs: 10g
- Fat: 14g

Vegan Stuffed Acorn Squash

Ingredients:

- 2 acorn squashes, halved and seeds removed
- 1 cup quinoa, cooked
- 1/2 cup black beans, drained and rinsed
- 1/4 cup cranberries
- 1/4 cup pecans, chopped

- 2 tbsp olive oil
- 1 tsp cumin
- Salt and pepper to taste

Instructions:

1. Preheat oven to 375°F (190°C).
2. Brush acorn squash halves with olive oil, salt, and pepper. Place cut-side down on a baking sheet and bake for 40-45 minutes.
3. In a bowl, mix cooked quinoa, black beans, cranberries, pecans, cumin, salt, and pepper.
4. Stuff each acorn squash half with the quinoa mixture.
5. Return to the oven and bake for another 10-15 minutes.

Nutritional Information (per serving):

- Calories: 350
- Protein: 10g
- Carbs: 50g
- Fat: 14g

7

Snack and Dessert Recipes

Healthy Snacking for PCOS

Snacking can be an important part of managing PCOS, as it helps maintain stable blood sugar levels and prevents overeating during meals. Opt for snacks that are high in protein, healthy fats, and fiber.

Guilt-Free Snack Ideas

- **Energy Balls**
- **Veggie Chips**
- **Yogurt Parfaits**

Delicious and Healthy Desserts

- **Sugar-Free Treats**
- **Fruit-Based Desserts**

Almond Butter Energy Balls

Ingredients:

- 1 cup rolled oats
- 1/2 cup almond butter
- 1/4 cup honey
- 1/4 cup flaxseeds

- 1/4 cup mini chocolate chips
- 1 tsp vanilla extract

Instructions:

1. In a large bowl, mix all ingredients until well combined.
2. Roll the mixture into small balls and place them on a baking sheet.
3. Refrigerate for at least 30 minutes before serving.

Nutritional Information (per serving - 2 balls):

- Calories: 200
- Protein: 6g
- Carbs: 20g
- Fat: 12g

Kale Chips

Ingredients:

- 1 bunch kale, washed and dried
- 1 tbsp olive oil
- 1/2 tsp sea salt

Instructions:

1. Preheat oven to 350°F (175°C).
2. Remove kale leaves from the stems and tear them into bite-sized pieces.
3. Toss kale with olive oil and sea salt.
4. Spread kale on a baking sheet in a single layer.
5. Bake for 10-15 minutes or until crispy.

Nutritional Information (per serving):

- Calories: 50
- Protein: 2g
- Carbs: 7g
- Fat: 2g

Greek Yogurt with Honey and Nuts

Ingredients:

- 1 cup Greek yogurt
- 1 tbsp honey
- 1/4 cup mixed nuts, chopped

Instructions:

1. Spoon Greek yogurt into a bowl.
2. Drizzle with honey and top with mixed nuts.

Nutritional Information (per serving):

- Calories: 250
- Protein: 15g
- Carbs: 20g
- Fat: 12g

Dark Chocolate Avocado Mousse

Ingredients:

- 2 ripe avocados
- 1/4 cup cocoa powder

- 1/4 cup honey
- 1 tsp vanilla extract
- A pinch of sea salt

Instructions:

1. In a food processor, blend avocados until smooth.
2. Add cocoa powder, honey, vanilla extract, and sea salt. Blend until well combined.
3. Spoon the mousse into serving bowls and refrigerate for at least 30 minutes before serving.

Nutritional Information (per serving):

- Calories: 200
- Protein: 3g
- Carbs: 25g
- Fat: 12g

Berry Smoothie Popsicles

Ingredients:

- 2 cups mixed berries
- 1 cup Greek yogurt
- 1/2 cup almond milk
- 1 tbsp honey

Instructions:

1. Blend all ingredients until smooth.
2. Pour the mixture into popsicle molds.
3. Freeze for at least 4 hours or until solid.

Nutritional Information (per serving):

- Calories: 100
- Protein: 5g
- Carbs: 20g
- Fat: 2g

Hummus and Veggie Sticks

Ingredients:

- 1 cup hummus
- 1 carrot, cut into sticks
- 1 cucumber, cut into sticks
- 1 bell pepper, cut into sticks

Instructions:

1. Arrange veggie sticks on a plate.
2. Serve with hummus for dipping.

Nutritional Information (per serving):

- Calories: 150
- Protein: 5g
- Carbs: 20g
- Fat: 8g

Spicy Roasted Chickpeas

Ingredients:

- 1 can chickpeas, drained and rinsed

- 1 tbsp olive oil
- 1 tsp paprika
- 1/2 tsp cayenne pepper
- 1/2 tsp garlic powder
- Salt to taste

Instructions:

1. Preheat oven to 400°F (200°C).
2. Toss chickpeas with olive oil and spices.
3. Spread chickpeas on a baking sheet in a single layer.
4. Roast for 20-25 minutes, stirring occasionally, until crispy.

Nutritional Information (per serving):

- Calories: 120
- Protein: 6g
- Carbs: 20g
- Fat: 4g

Peanut Butter Banana Bites

Ingredients:

- 2 bananas, sliced
- 1/4 cup peanut butter
- 1/4 cup dark chocolate chips

Instructions:

1. Spread peanut butter on half of the banana slices.
2. Top with the remaining banana slices to make sandwiches.
3. Melt dark chocolate chips and drizzle over the banana sandwiches.

4. Freeze for at least 30 minutes before serving.

Nutritional Information (per serving - 2 bites):

- Calories: 150
- Protein: 3g
- Carbs: 25g
- Fat: 8g

Strawberry Chia Pudding

Ingredients:

- 1 cup almond milk
- 1/4 cup chia seeds
- 1 cup strawberries, chopped
- 1 tbsp honey

Instructions:

1. In a bowl, mix almond milk, chia seeds, and honey.
2. Stir in chopped strawberries.
3. Refrigerate overnight or for at least 4 hours until thickened.

Nutritional Information (per serving):

- Calories: 200
- Protein: 5g
- Carbs: 30g
- Fat: 8g

Apple Nachos with Almond Butter

Ingredients:

- 2 apples, sliced
- 2 tbsp almond butter
- 1 tbsp mini chocolate chips
- 1 tbsp shredded coconut

Instructions:

1. Arrange apple slices on a plate.
2. Drizzle with almond butter.
3. Sprinkle with mini chocolate chips and shredded coconut.

Nutritional Information (per serving):

- Calories: 250
- Protein: 4g
- Carbs: 35g
- Fat: 12g

Cinnamon Roasted Almonds

Ingredients:

- 2 cups raw almonds
- 2 tbsp maple syrup
- 1 tsp cinnamon
- A pinch of sea salt

Instructions:

1. Preheat oven to 350°F (175°C).
2. Toss almonds with maple syrup, cinnamon, and sea salt.
3. Spread almonds on a baking sheet in a single layer.
4. Bake for 10-15 minutes, stirring occasionally.

Nutritional Information (per serving - 1/4 cup):

- Calories: 200
- Protein: 6g
- Carbs: 10g
- Fat: 16g

Coconut Macaroons

Ingredients:

- 2 cups shredded coconut
- 1/4 cup honey
- 2 egg whites
- 1 tsp vanilla extract

Instructions:

1. Preheat oven to 325°F (160°C).
2. In a bowl, mix shredded coconut, honey, egg whites, and vanilla extract.
3. Scoop small mounds of the mixture onto a baking sheet lined with parchment paper.
4. Bake for 15-20 minutes or until golden brown.

Nutritional Information (per serving - 2 macaroons):

- Calories: 150

- Protein: 2g
- Carbs: 20g
- Fat: 8g

Pumpkin Spice Protein Bars

Ingredients:

- 1 cup rolled oats
- 1/2 cup pumpkin puree
- 1/4 cup protein powder
- 1/4 cup almond butter
- 2 tbsp honey
- 1 tsp pumpkin pie spice

Instructions:

1. In a large bowl, mix all ingredients until well combined.
2. Press the mixture into a baking dish lined with parchment paper.
3. Refrigerate for at least 1 hour before cutting into bars.

Nutritional Information (per serving - 1 bar):

- Calories: 200
- Protein: 8g
- Carbs: 25g
- Fat: 8g

Carrot Cake Energy Balls

Ingredients:

- 1 cup rolled oats

- 1/2 cup grated carrots
- 1/4 cup almond butter
- 1/4 cup honey
- 1/4 cup shredded coconut
- 1 tsp cinnamon

Instructions:

1. In a large bowl, mix all ingredients until well combined.
2. Roll the mixture into small balls and place them on a baking sheet.
3. Refrigerate for at least 30 minutes before serving.

Nutritional Information (per serving - 2 balls):

- Calories: 200
- Protein: 4g
- Carbs: 25g
- Fat: 10g

Mixed Berry Salad

Ingredients:

- 1 cup strawberries, sliced
- 1 cup blueberries
- 1 cup raspberries
- 1 cup blackberries
- 1 tbsp honey
- 1 tbsp lemon juice

Instructions:

1. In a large bowl, mix all berries.

2. Drizzle with honey and lemon juice. Toss to combine.

Nutritional Information (per serving):

- Calories: 100
- Protein: 2g
- Carbs: 25g
- Fat: 1g

Chocolate-Covered Strawberries

Ingredients:

- 1 cup dark chocolate chips
- 1 tbsp coconut oil
- 1 pint strawberries

Instructions:

1. In a microwave-safe bowl, melt dark chocolate chips and coconut oil in 30-second intervals, stirring until smooth.
2. Dip each strawberry into the melted chocolate and place them on a baking sheet lined with parchment paper.
3. Refrigerate for at least 30 minutes before serving.

Nutritional Information (per serving - 4 strawberries):

- Calories: 150
- Protein: 2g
- Carbs: 20g
- Fat: 8g

Raspberry Lemon Sorbet

Ingredients:

- 2 cups raspberries
- 1/2 cup lemon juice
- 1/2 cup honey
- 1 cup water

Instructions:

1. In a blender, combine raspberries, lemon juice, honey, and water. Blend until smooth.
2. Pour the mixture into a shallow dish and freeze for at least 4 hours, stirring occasionally.

Nutritional Information (per serving):

- Calories: 100
- Protein: 1g
- Carbs: 25g
- Fat: 0g

No-Bake Coconut Bars

Ingredients:

- 2 cups shredded coconut
- 1/2 cup coconut oil, melted
- 1/4 cup honey
- 1 tsp vanilla extract

Instructions:

1. In a bowl, mix shredded coconut, coconut oil, honey, and vanilla extract until well combined.
2. Press the mixture into a baking dish lined with parchment paper.
3. Refrigerate for at least 1 hour before cutting into bars.

Nutritional Information (per serving - 1 bar):

- Calories: 200
- Protein: 2g
- Carbs: 10g
- Fat: 18g

Oatmeal Cookies

Ingredients:

- 1 cup rolled oats
- 1/2 cup almond flour
- 1/4 cup coconut oil, melted
- 1/4 cup honey
- 1 tsp vanilla extract
- 1/2 tsp baking soda
- 1/2 cup raisins

Instructions:

1. Preheat oven to 350°F (175°C).
2. In a large bowl, mix all ingredients until well combined.
3. Drop spoonfuls of the mixture onto a baking sheet lined with parchment paper.
4. Bake for 10-12 minutes or until golden brown.

Nutritional Information (per serving - 2 cookies):

- Calories: 150
- Protein: 3g
- Carbs: 20g
- Fat: 8g

Mango Coconut Chia Pudding

Ingredients:

- 1 cup almond milk
- 1/4 cup chia seeds
- 1/2 cup mango, diced
- 1 tbsp shredded coconut
- 1 tbsp honey

Instructions:

1. In a bowl, mix almond milk, chia seeds, and honey.
2. Stir in diced mango.
3. Refrigerate overnight or for at least 4 hours until thickened.
4. Top with shredded coconut before serving.

Nutritional Information (per serving):

- Calories: 200
- Protein: 4g
- Carbs: 30g
- Fat: 8g

8

Meal Plans and Shopping Lists

Weekly Meal Plans

Having a meal plan can make managing PCOS and insulin resistance much easier. Here are sample weekly meal plans that cater to different dietary needs, along with tips for adjusting them based on individual preferences.

Sample Meal Plan 1: Balanced Diet

Monday

- **Breakfast:** Green Smoothie Bowl
- **Lunch:** Mediterranean Chickpea Salad
- **Dinner:** Baked Lemon Herb Chicken with a side of roasted vegetables
- **Snack:** Almond Butter Energy Balls

Tuesday

- **Breakfast:** Cinnamon Apple Overnight Oats
- **Lunch:** Grilled Chicken Caesar Wrap
- **Dinner:** Garlic Shrimp Stir-Fry with brown rice
- **Snack:** Greek Yogurt with Honey and Nuts

Wednesday

- **Breakfast:** Veggie-Packed Egg Muffins
- **Lunch:** Quinoa and Black Bean Salad
- **Dinner:** Beef and Broccoli with quinoa
- **Snack:** Kale Chips

Thursday

- **Breakfast:** Avocado Toast with a Twist
- **Lunch:** Turkey Avocado Club
- **Dinner:** Spaghetti Squash Bolognese
- **Snack:** Dark Chocolate Avocado Mousse

Friday

- **Breakfast:** Chia Seed Pudding with Berries
- **Lunch:** Thai Peanut Noodle Bowl
- **Dinner:** Herb-Crusted Salmon with a side salad
- **Snack:** Berry Smoothie Popsicles

Saturday

- **Breakfast:** Spinach and Feta Breakfast Wrap
- **Lunch:** Shrimp and Avocado Salad
- **Dinner:** Veggie-Packed Chili
- **Snack:** Hummus and Veggie Sticks

Sunday

- **Breakfast:** Greek Yogurt Parfait
- **Lunch:** Vegan Buddha Bowl
- **Dinner:** Pesto Chicken Bake with quinoa
- **Snack:** Spicy Roasted Chickpeas

Sample Meal Plan 2: Low-Carb Diet

Monday

- **Breakfast:** Almond Flour Pancakes
- **Lunch:** Spinach and Quinoa Stuffed Peppers
- **Dinner:** Lemon Garlic Tilapia with cauliflower rice
- **Snack:** Peanut Butter Banana Bites

Tuesday

- **Breakfast:** Tofu Scramble
- **Lunch:** Chicken and Veggie Stir-Fry
- **Dinner:** Thai Green Curry with zoodles
- **Snack:** Cinnamon Roasted Almonds

Wednesday

- **Breakfast:** Quinoa Breakfast Bowl
- **Lunch:** Tuna Salad Lettuce Wraps
- **Dinner:** Turkey Meatballs with Zoodles
- **Snack:** Coconut Macaroons

Thursday

- **Breakfast:** Breakfast Burrito
- **Lunch:** Falafel Bowl
- **Dinner:** Balsamic Glazed Pork Chops with a side salad
- **Snack:** Pumpkin Spice Protein Bars

Friday

- **Breakfast:** Protein-Packed Smoothie

- **Lunch:** Zucchini Noodles with Pesto
- **Dinner:** Chicken Fajita Bowl
- **Snack:** Carrot Cake Energy Balls

Saturday

- **Breakfast:** Sweet Potato Hash
- **Lunch:** Spaghetti Squash Pad Thai
- **Dinner:** Mediterranean Lamb Stew
- **Snack:** Mixed Berry Salad

Sunday

- **Breakfast:** Mushroom Omelette
- **Lunch:** Roasted Veggie Wrap
- **Dinner:** Stuffed Bell Peppers
- **Snack:** Chocolate-Covered Strawberries

Adjusting Meal Plans Based on Individual Preferences

- **Vegetarian Options:** Substitute animal proteins with plant-based alternatives like tofu, tempeh, lentils, and beans.
- **Vegan Options:** Use vegan alternatives like plant-based milk, yogurt, and cheese.
- **Gluten-Free Options:** Ensure all grains and flours are gluten-free, such as using gluten-free oats and quinoa.
- **Pescatarian Options:** Incorporate more seafood-based meals, such as shrimp, salmon, and tilapia.

Shopping Lists

Sample Shopping List for Balanced Diet Meal Plan

Produce:

- Spinach (2 bunches)
- Avocado (5)
- Bananas (4)
- Apples (3)
- Berries (assorted, 4 cups)
- Cherry tomatoes (3 cups)
- Cucumber (3)
- Bell peppers (5)
- Broccoli (2 crowns)
- Zucchini (4)
- Carrots (6)
- Onions (4)
- Garlic (2 bulbs)
- Lemon (4)
- Lime (2)
- Sweet potatoes (4)
- Mixed greens (2 bags)
- Romaine lettuce (1 head)

Proteins:

- Chicken breasts (8)
- Shrimp (2 lbs)
- Ground turkey (1 lb)
- Salmon fillets (4)
- Tilapia fillets (4)
- Turkey breast slices (1 pack)

- Eggs (2 dozen)
- Greek yogurt (4 cups)
- Hummus (1 cup)
- Black beans (2 cans)
- Chickpeas (2 cans)
- Tuna (2 cans)
- Almond butter (1 jar)
- Almond milk (1 carton)

Grains and Nuts:

- Rolled oats (1 bag)
- Quinoa (1 bag)
- Whole wheat tortillas (1 pack)
- Brown rice (1 bag)
- Panko breadcrumbs (1 box)
- Parmesan cheese (1 block)
- Mini chocolate chips (1 bag)
- Mixed nuts (1 bag)
- Flaxseeds (1 bag)
- Chia seeds (1 bag)

Condiments and Spices:

- Olive oil (1 bottle)
- Soy sauce (1 bottle)
- Basil pesto (1 jar)
- BBQ sauce (1 bottle)
- Tahini (1 jar)
- Maple syrup (1 bottle)
- Honey (1 bottle)
- Almond butter (1 jar)
- Coconut oil (1 jar)

- Cocoa powder (1 bag)
- Various spices (cinnamon, paprika, cumin, turmeric, chili powder, oregano, thyme, basil, coriander, sea salt, black pepper, garlic powder, red pepper flakes)

Other:

- Whole grain bread (1 loaf)
- Whole grain pasta (1 box)
- Dark chocolate chips (1 bag)
- Coconut flakes (1 bag)
- Canned diced tomatoes (4 cans)
- Canned coconut milk (2 cans)
- Vegetable broth (1 box)

Tips for Efficient Grocery Shopping

1. **Organize Your List by Section:** Group items by produce, dairy, meat, grains, and pantry to make shopping quicker.
2. **Buy in Bulk:** Purchase non-perishable items like oats, nuts, seeds, and grains in bulk to save money.
3. **Use Fresh and Frozen Produce:** Fresh produce is great for immediate use, while frozen fruits and vegetables can be used in smoothies, stir-fries, and soups.
4. **Check for Sales and Coupons:** Look for discounts and use coupons to save on your grocery bill.
5. **Stick to the List:** Avoid impulse buying by sticking to your shopping list, ensuring you get only what you need for your meal plans.

9

Meal Plans and Shopping Lists

Weekly Meal Plans

Having a meal plan can make managing PCOS and insulin resistance much easier. Here are sample weekly meal plans that cater to different dietary needs, along with tips for adjusting them based on individual preferences.

Sample Meal Plan 1: Balanced Diet

Monday

- **Breakfast:** Green Smoothie Bowl
- **Lunch:** Mediterranean Chickpea Salad
- **Dinner:** Baked Lemon Herb Chicken with a side of roasted vegetables
- **Snack:** Almond Butter Energy Balls

Tuesday

- **Breakfast:** Cinnamon Apple Overnight Oats
- **Lunch:** Grilled Chicken Caesar Wrap
- **Dinner:** Garlic Shrimp Stir-Fry with brown rice
- **Snack:** Greek Yogurt with Honey and Nuts

Wednesday

- **Breakfast:** Veggie-Packed Egg Muffins
- **Lunch:** Quinoa and Black Bean Salad
- **Dinner:** Beef and Broccoli with quinoa
- **Snack:** Kale Chips

Thursday

- **Breakfast:** Avocado Toast with a Twist
- **Lunch:** Turkey Avocado Club
- **Dinner:** Spaghetti Squash Bolognese
- **Snack:** Dark Chocolate Avocado Mousse

Friday

- **Breakfast:** Chia Seed Pudding with Berries
- **Lunch:** Thai Peanut Noodle Bowl
- **Dinner:** Herb-Crusted Salmon with a side salad
- **Snack:** Berry Smoothie Popsicles

Saturday

- **Breakfast:** Spinach and Feta Breakfast Wrap
- **Lunch:** Shrimp and Avocado Salad
- **Dinner:** Veggie-Packed Chili
- **Snack:** Hummus and Veggie Sticks

Sunday

- **Breakfast:** Greek Yogurt Parfait
- **Lunch:** Vegan Buddha Bowl
- **Dinner:** Pesto Chicken Bake with quinoa
- **Snack:** Spicy Roasted Chickpeas

Sample Meal Plan 2: Low-Carb Diet

Monday

- **Breakfast:** Almond Flour Pancakes
- **Lunch:** Spinach and Quinoa Stuffed Peppers
- **Dinner:** Lemon Garlic Tilapia with cauliflower rice
- **Snack:** Peanut Butter Banana Bites

Tuesday

- **Breakfast:** Tofu Scramble
- **Lunch:** Chicken and Veggie Stir-Fry
- **Dinner:** Thai Green Curry with zoodles
- **Snack:** Cinnamon Roasted Almonds

Wednesday

- **Breakfast:** Quinoa Breakfast Bowl
- **Lunch:** Tuna Salad Lettuce Wraps
- **Dinner:** Turkey Meatballs with Zoodles
- **Snack:** Coconut Macaroons

Thursday

- **Breakfast:** Breakfast Burrito
- **Lunch:** Falafel Bowl
- **Dinner:** Balsamic Glazed Pork Chops with a side salad
- **Snack:** Pumpkin Spice Protein Bars

Friday

- **Breakfast:** Protein-Packed Smoothie

- **Lunch:** Zucchini Noodles with Pesto
- **Dinner:** Chicken Fajita Bowl
- **Snack:** Carrot Cake Energy Balls

Saturday

- **Breakfast:** Sweet Potato Hash
- **Lunch:** Spaghetti Squash Pad Thai
- **Dinner:** Mediterranean Lamb Stew
- **Snack:** Mixed Berry Salad

Sunday

- **Breakfast:** Mushroom Omelette
- **Lunch:** Roasted Veggie Wrap
- **Dinner:** Stuffed Bell Peppers
- **Snack:** Chocolate-Covered Strawberries

Adjusting Meal Plans Based on Individual Preferences

- **Vegetarian Options:** Substitute animal proteins with plant-based alternatives like tofu, tempeh, lentils, and beans.
- **Vegan Options:** Use vegan alternatives like plant-based milk, yogurt, and cheese.
- **Gluten-Free Options:** Ensure all grains and flours are gluten-free, such as using gluten-free oats and quinoa.
- **Pescatarian Options:** Incorporate more seafood-based meals, such as shrimp, salmon, and tilapia.

Shopping Lists

Sample Shopping List for Balanced Diet Meal Plan

Produce:

- Spinach (2 bunches)
- Avocado (5)
- Bananas (4)
- Apples (3)
- Berries (assorted, 4 cups)
- Cherry tomatoes (3 cups)
- Cucumber (3)
- Bell peppers (5)
- Broccoli (2 crowns)
- Zucchini (4)
- Carrots (6)
- Onions (4)
- Garlic (2 bulbs)
- Lemon (4)
- Lime (2)
- Sweet potatoes (4)
- Mixed greens (2 bags)
- Romaine lettuce (1 head)

Proteins:

- Chicken breasts (8)
- Shrimp (2 lbs)
- Ground turkey (1 lb)
- Salmon fillets (4)
- Tilapia fillets (4)
- Turkey breast slices (1 pack)

- Eggs (2 dozen)
- Greek yogurt (4 cups)
- Hummus (1 cup)
- Black beans (2 cans)
- Chickpeas (2 cans)
- Tuna (2 cans)
- Almond butter (1 jar)
- Almond milk (1 carton)

Grains and Nuts:

- Rolled oats (1 bag)
- Quinoa (1 bag)
- Whole wheat tortillas (1 pack)
- Brown rice (1 bag)
- Panko breadcrumbs (1 box)
- Parmesan cheese (1 block)
- Mini chocolate chips (1 bag)
- Mixed nuts (1 bag)
- Flaxseeds (1 bag)
- Chia seeds (1 bag)

Condiments and Spices:

- Olive oil (1 bottle)
- Soy sauce (1 bottle)
- Basil pesto (1 jar)
- BBQ sauce (1 bottle)
- Tahini (1 jar)
- Maple syrup (1 bottle)
- Honey (1 bottle)
- Almond butter (1 jar)
- Coconut oil (1 jar)

- Cocoa powder (1 bag)
- Various spices (cinnamon, paprika, cumin, turmeric, chili powder, oregano, thyme, basil, coriander, sea salt, black pepper, garlic powder, red pepper flakes)

Other:

- Whole grain bread (1 loaf)
- Whole grain pasta (1 box)
- Dark chocolate chips (1 bag)
- Coconut flakes (1 bag)
- Canned diced tomatoes (4 cans)
- Canned coconut milk (2 cans)
- Vegetable broth (1 box)

Tips for Efficient Grocery Shopping

1. **Organize Your List by Section:** Group items by produce, dairy, meat, grains, and pantry to make shopping quicker.
2. **Buy in Bulk:** Purchase non-perishable items like oats, nuts, seeds, and grains in bulk to save money.
3. **Use Fresh and Frozen Produce:** Fresh produce is great for immediate use, while frozen fruits and vegetables can be used in smoothies, stir-fries, and soups.
4. **Check for Sales and Coupons:** Look for discounts and use coupons to save on your grocery bill.
5. **Stick to the List:** Avoid impulse buying by sticking to your shopping list, ensuring you get only what you need for your meal plans.

10

Success Stories and Testimonials

Real-Life Examples

Sharing real-life success stories can be incredibly motivating for readers. These stories not only provide inspiration but also practical tips and insights on managing PCOS through diet and lifestyle changes. Here are a few success stories from women who have successfully managed their PCOS with the help of this cookbook's principles.

Success Story 1: Sarah's Journey to Balance

Background: Sarah was diagnosed with PCOS at the age of 25. She struggled with weight gain, irregular periods, and acne. Despite trying various diets, nothing seemed to work.

The Transformation: Sarah discovered the importance of managing insulin resistance through diet. She started meal prepping using recipes from this cookbook, focusing on balanced meals with lean proteins, healthy fats, and complex carbohydrates. Over six months, she lost 20 pounds, her periods became regular, and her skin cleared up.

Tips from Sarah:

- **Consistency is Key:** Stick to your meal prep routine to avoid falling back into unhealthy habits.

- **Experiment with Recipes:** Don't be afraid to tweak recipes to suit your taste buds.
- **Stay Hydrated:** Drink plenty of water throughout the day to help with digestion and overall health.

Success Story 2: Emma's Path to Wellness

Background: Emma had been dealing with PCOS symptoms since her teens. She faced challenges with excessive hair growth, fatigue, and mood swings. Traditional treatments provided little relief.

The Transformation: Emma decided to take control of her PCOS through diet and exercise. She incorporated the recipes from this cookbook into her daily routine, ensuring she had a variety of meals to keep things interesting. Within four months, she noticed a significant reduction in her symptoms and an overall improvement in her energy levels.

Tips from Emma:

- **Plan Ahead:** Make a weekly meal plan to ensure you have all the ingredients you need.
- **Find Support:** Join a community or support group to share experiences and stay motivated.
- **Celebrate Small Wins:** Acknowledge and celebrate small achievements along the way.

Success Story 3: Olivia's Lifestyle Change

Background: Olivia struggled with PCOS-related infertility for years. After several unsuccessful treatments, she decided to explore dietary changes as a natural approach to managing her condition.

The Transformation: By following the insulin resistance diet and using the recipes in this cookbook, Olivia was able to regulate her blood sugar levels and improve her overall health. Within a year, she successfully conceived and continued to use the principles of this cookbook to maintain a healthy pregnancy.

Tips from Olivia:

- **Keep it Simple:** Start with easy recipes and gradually try more complex ones.
- **Be Patient:** Dietary changes take time to show results, so stay patient and persistent.
- **Include Your Family:** Get your family involved in meal prepping and cooking to make it a fun, shared activity.

Tips and Advice from Real Women

In addition to sharing their stories, these women have practical advice and motivational tips to help you on your journey.

- **Stay Positive:** Focus on the positive changes you're making rather than the challenges you face.
- **Track Your Progress:** Keep a journal to track your meals, symptoms, and progress over time.
- **Seek Professional Guidance:** Consult with a healthcare professional or nutritionist to tailor the diet to your specific needs.

Community and Support

Building a support network can make a significant difference in your journey to manage PCOS. Here are some resources to help you find community and support:

- **Online Support Groups:** Join forums and social media groups dedicated to PCOS management and healthy eating.
- **Local Meetups:** Look for local groups or events focused on women's health and wellness.

- **Professional Support:** Work with a dietitian, nutritionist, or healthcare provider who specializes in PCOS.

Conclusion

Final Thoughts and Encouragement

Managing PCOS can be challenging, but with the right tools and support, you can take control of your health. Remember that every small step counts and that consistency and patience are key. This cookbook is designed to make the journey easier by providing you with delicious, nutritious recipes that support insulin sensitivity and overall well-being.

Additional Resources

For further reading and support, here are some recommended resources:

- **Books:** "The PCOS Plan" by Dr. Jason Fung, "PCOS Diet for Beginners" by Jennifer Koslo
- **Websites:** PCOS Challenge (pcoschallenge.org), PCOS Nutrition Center (pcosnutrition.com)
- **Support Groups:** Find local and online support groups through platforms like Meetup or Facebook.

Final Review and Compilation

To ensure the content is coherent and consistent, we'll compile all the chapters and review the entire cookbook. This includes:

1. **Introduction**
2. **Understanding PCOS and Insulin Resistance**
3. **Meal Prep Basics**

4. **Breakfast Recipes**
5. **Lunch Recipes**
6. **Dinner Recipes**
7. **Snack and Dessert Recipes**
8. **Success Stories and Testimonials**